Oxygen Yoga

Handbook

Ellis & Cito

authorHOUSE®

AuthorHouse™
1663 Liberty Drive, Suite 200
Bloomington, IN 47403
www.authorhouse.com
Phone: 1-800-839-8640

First published by AuthorHouse   10/23/2008

ISBN: 978-1-4389-1276-9 (sc)

Printed in the United States of America
Bloomington, Indiana

This book is printed on acid-free paper.

The Oxygen Yoga Handbook

21ST CENTURY, AMERICAN   FITNESS PROGAM

A warm-up, introductory manual for guiding the novice into the full Oxygen Yoga: Pure and Simple program

by

Barbara Ellis and Lisa Cito

For Lisa Cito's husband, Savino,

Her parents John and Josie and to Barbara's father, George Cvetkovich

The wind beneath our wings

. . . At night, I open the window and ask

the moon to come and press its

face against mine.

Breathe into me.

Close the language-door and

open the love window.

The moon

won't use the door, only the window.

From the Coleman Barks Translations of Rumi

Contents

A PRELUDE TO YOUR SPIRITUAL PATH . xiii

1   Breathing and Rapid Aging 1

2   What's a Brain got to do with it?.............. 7

3   Pollution and the Air We Breathe 17

4   Letting the Body Quiet the Mind 27

5   Oxygenized Yoga Changes Being Alive .. 37

6   The First Step Begins Now 47

7   The Promise of a Body Full of Oxygen .. 71

8   Today is Spa Day 81

RAISING WIND HORSE 89

ABOUT THE AUTHORS 101

A PRELUDE TO YOUR SPIRITUAL PATH

You are standing at a threshold, a remarkable portal through which you can step into the rest of your life with a sense of renewal, a brand new relationship with yourself, your loved ones, and the world around you. This new era is not just words, not just more hype, not wishful thinking but the actual truth that you can feel, can feel immediately, can feel with your entire body.

The mind can dodge the truth, can be slippery and confusing, and can overwhelm us with thinking. It is not always the place to look for a valid appraisal of what is taking place. But the body never fails us with her clear messages.

When we learn to listen to our bodies, they will never fail to communicate with us but will offer up their clear and vibrant messages without a moment's hesitation. This booklet; the workshops; the textbook, *Oxygen Yoga Pure & Simple;* the enhanced liveliness; the natural wealth of gaining full, deep, vital, energy-giving breath; all of the gifts of 0_2 work become the foundation for the Spiritual Path.

Moving into the 21st Century, we are at an amazing pinnacle in human history. The new millennium has opened its floodgates with a fabulous array of events that are rapidly drawing us toward the next phase in human growth as moths are drawn to flame.

We all know about the difficult situations facing us on this gorgeous, little, blue planet; but, how often are we reminded that we now have a great opportunity directly in the palm of our hands. In this new century we have distilled all the great teachings that have come down to us since the initial stages of human understanding, since the incubation of spiritual training somewhere after the last ice age, have fine tuned them into simple forms. We don't need to sit around hoping that on some far-distant day we might, that just maybe, we can possibly be released into the Enlightened Mind.

No, we can now use Oxygen Yoga as a base platform and through the stillness created in our minds via the roadmap created by Yoga and meditations natural quieting of mental chatter, learn to relax, to open to the eternal moment, the never-ending dance of the universe that surrounds us at all times, to become one with our environs and allow happiness of fill our every cell. We do not have to limit the infusion of O_2 or the stretching to theory. We can feel them as we release ourselves from corporate products and adapt to a natural beauty treatment.

Use this handbook to step right through the portal of all that has come down to us from the last few decades of the 20th Century, to step through into the fusion of the knowledge of great teachers like Gandhi, his showing us how to relax into the profound happiness of finding peace in our hearts in the midst of the most violent of opposition.

As this handbook entrenches your understanding of Oxygen Yoga, you will begin to see how important your breath is and become aware of how badly we are deprived of our most important toehold on our lives, oxygen. The Dali Lama began his life with a super abundance of oxygen in the Himalayas. Day in and day out, the pure, crisp air that he and all of the original Tibetan teachers breathed, brought them rapidly into the sleek, diamantine awareness for which they are so renowned.

When we hear the venerable teachers of Tibet speak, we can feel the oxygen based awareness that provided the clarity of the original teachings. Now, we don't need to go to Tibet to enjoy this birthright that all of us deserve—Oxygen Yoga begins to take you to the threshold of clarity with your first in-breath. As you exhale, you will need more, and the new breath will fill your entire brain, your whole body with properly oxygenated blood. It is no secret how healthy looking, how beautiful the skin is of people like the Tibetans who breathe huge amounts of O_2. Oxygen Yoga makes the body radiant.

The miracle is that you don't have to study with teachers for decades on end wondering if you are okay, if you should look up Dr. Phil for consultation, if you will be stuck feeling lost and confused all your life. No, you can feel your way directly into enlightened mind via the veracity of knowing your own body. Oxygen Yoga presents you with pure, simple visceral understanding. As we open to listening to our bodies, becoming more and more aware of them, we understand fully that the body does not lie. Only the mind takes off on misinformation and launches our all-consuming mental chatter, creating a cluttered mentality.

You will be using this booklet to begin to give your mind the big, spacious sense of calm that Oxygen Yoga provides, and then with skill and more rapidly than you might think, you will use your findings here to progress into the teachings in the full textbook—*Oxygen Yoga: Pure & Simple*—and proceed to take the courses and to fill in the blanks of your understanding

It is all actually quite simple. Thousands of years back in history, when the teachings arose, the children were a very important part of executing the daily tasks required for existence. The elders lived close, entwined within the family unit and were listened to for sage advice. The fruits of a family's labor were very precious due to the vast effort required for production—and, there was a huge abundance of simple, pure oxygen in the air these ancestors breathed.

Needless to say, the early period was a much different time than these centuries in which we are now living. The origin of the great spiritual teachings required the implantation of deep concerns about being banished if we did not pay attention—though they were built not on fear but learning to understand what behaviors free us in life and what habits bind us to our egos.

But now, in this 'Brave New World' we live at the speed of electrons and that is how we must move toward the Enlightened Mind. You will find that this handbook can be the prelude to a deeply rewarding spiritual life. As you move from the handbook, into the textbook, *Oxygen Yoga Pure & Simple,* and begin the Oxygen Yoga practice, the involvement brings you face to face with feeling the true clarity of those first teachers. Deep understanding requires the same levels of oxygen which they enjoyed in order to experience our own beings at their fullest.

The following eight chapters of the handbook will open your eyes to the new wave of teaching and provide a base for all of your spiritual studies. Many of you will see already the ultimate importance of quieting our unending mental chatter with the subtle body control of Yoga movements while enhancing our beings with oxygen.

Those of you with this clarity can mover right straight through to the end of the handbook and utilize the RAISING WIND HORSE section to move on into your new life of Oxygen Yoga. First you will pick up the text book—*Oxygen Yoga Pure & Simple.* You will then proceed to a center and take up the practice. The tapes and CDs will be of help as you proceed along your spirit journey.

With warm regards,
Barbara and Lisa

CHAPTER 1

BREATHING AND RAPID AGING

We can live for quite some time without food. We have seen it with the long fasts of prophets and socially conscious protestors, over a month with nothing more than some orange juice in water. The need for water, though it is pressing, leaves us a bit of time to search for a supply before we perish.

* * * OGA NOTE ***

If you already understand where we are going, you can pass this handbook on to friends and order your copy of Oxygen Yoga Pure & Simple right now. Just type www. oxygenyogabook.com **into the address line on your computer and get it now.**

Sign up for a beginner's class immediately and never look back.

On the street you are at the mercy of manufacturing plants, the construction industry and trucks and autos. The only thing we can do about this pickle is to use the internet and our vote to take power away from the top shareholders of the corporations who own the politicians with their lobbyists. All of the seemingly uncontrollable issues are rampant because the politicians are dupes, they are owned by the contributions of the majority stockholders who pummel our corporations into mindless greed. The bottom line of cash flow has become the only part of the majority of businesses that is of any importance. We are enjoying some token changes with the new wave of green, but don't let anyone lull you to sleep with green marketing propaganda—our lungs are brutalized every moment, 24/7.

Oga is one thing, another wonderful thing—as well as cleaning up your home and place of business—by which you can make a true and immediate difference for your lungs, your skin tone, your face and so on.

The practice of Oxygen Yoga is a form that takes the practitioner deep inside, slows the mind down, and allows a person to know the breath fully. In the process, one comes to the conscious realization that we need to become intimate with our entire, fabulous process of breathing.

We created Oxygen Yoga (Oga) to help each and every one of us learn to remember our breath, to be tuned in fully to the urgency, to undertake the filling of our lungs completely within moments after an exhale. To enjoy an intake that can be felt clear down to the bone-plate of the pelvis.

* * * OGA NOTE * * *

Be sure to find an architect who has a good reference list of people to call for whom she or he has created non-toxic, clean air homes.

The difference for your lungs in your toxin-free home will be like leaving a restaurant in an area where smoking is allowed—you will feel invigorated throughout your entire being, inside and out.

How few of us know our breath intimately, know how we can use it fully, right there in every moment of our lives in the moment to help us release stressful emotions and to generate a full spread of an extended, loving, wholesome, vigorous, rousing, joyous, a truly fulfilling life. History is ripe with insightful teachings about the use of our wondrous respiratory system.

The word has begun to spread in modern times—just look at how many public places and people's homes is smoke free. It is becoming more and more obvious that as we try to fight for clean air, trying to become a GREEN society, grow more alert, we understand just how seriously important it is to have corporations help in this quest to reduce smog and dangerous chemicals contaminating our air.

Real attention is now being paid to our breathing. The time keeping mechanisms that work with one's entire body and set up the ticking clock that takes us into old age and on to the great change, the magical shift from life into our deaths are always at work. But there are things that speed the tick-tock up. Now, the avant-garde researchers are deeply involved in reviewing the telomeres—the area where repetitive DNA chromosomes work with aging and cancer--and they are comparing them to a specially designed string of pearls, DNA suspended at the end of chromosomes, strings of magic, which get shorter with every cell division. The data is streaming in, the research is moving along at a furious pace all round the globe. Every day it appears to be more and more likely that oxygen can not only make our lives more vital but can actually prolong them.

* * * OGA NOTE * * *

More and more, those deep researchers all around the world who are studying oxygen are coming to the same understanding. A healthy, clean, well-balance intake of this element essential to the existence of human beings can enhance the quality of a life, work with the aging process, keep the skin fresh and radiant. And, the scarcity of air well infused with O_2 is definitely impairment to enjoying a fully charged life. Oxygen Yoga was designed to aid people with this global catastrophe.

The knowledge of the great balancing power of stretching our bodies is very wide spread—certain forms of meticulous stretching are correspondent with yoga forms found from the roof tops of Tibet, all the way down through India, and out across Asia through Taoist Martial Arts temples in the most sacred caves of China.

These movements, whether found in the common stretching a person does instinctively when arising from a long trip in a car, or, the most guarded traditions found in the crevices circling the Fertile Crescent, accelerate the intake of oxygen into the blood stream and hasten the supply of robust, oxygen laden cells to the brain.

THE INTAKE OF OXYGEN IS BEING RESEARCHED AND APPLIED IN MANY WAYS

• Oxygen and cancer—hyperbaric—or increased oxygen pressure for treatment of cancers.

• The effects of a lack of oxygen on our minds; free radicals reacting with oxygen and triggering damage to the mitochondria—the power engines in our cells.

• Our skin, our faces our general radiance is spilling over from the many findings in the labs, straight into spas all over the world.With Oxygen Yoga, we have introduced a wonderful new form for enhancing the supply of O2 in the blood stream. The treatment brings the tools of yogins and yoginis throughout time—with their long, healthy lives and that extraordinary glow of youthfulness even in their eighties and nineties that have been a part of their legend—home to the everyday person.

CHAPTER 2

WHAT'S A BRAIN GOT TO DO WITH IT

There are periods in our lives when we look out on the world and see our loved ones, the trees, the lush fields, the valleys, the sky so blue and compassionate in its immensity—times when we actually see rather than just glancing at what surrounds us and zipping on past.

During those times when our minds are not spinning around, when we are not just wasting time doing something vacuous like slavishly watching TV or passing judgments on those around us, there are actually times when our eyes may stop for a moment, our mental chatter melts away and we enjoy a look, a long, slow and real look at the world. Those moments, which all of us have known here and there, are a brief taste of the feeling of enlightened mind. Returning to the busy parts of life, the mind kicks right back in and jerks us into the circle of endless— and almost entirely, negative chatter. We stay so wrapped up in our mental babble that we barely notice our physical surroundings, let alone what is going on inside.

At the same time that our minds hammer us with pointless chatter, our beings perform an unfathomable array of tasks that are absolutely required for the possibility of existence in this human form. The process of using air from our breathing alone is completely amazing. Thinking about the many things oxygen is doing and of the untold numbers of other activities that are required in order to stay alive, it is easy to feel deep appreciation for the brilliant intelligence of our bodies.

When we think of all the vitamins, the neurons, the gasses, the mineral compounds, clusters of atoms swirling around, breaking down, forming new compounds, it can all sound so scientific, so far removed from the wonderful clouds, the trees, the song of our hearts. And yet, the science is not separate inside us—as the wise ones have told us since before recorded history, all things are totally one.

Even while we are working through our deepest understanding in the dream world, chatting with friends, washing the dishes, every beat of our lives begins, and melts into the next event right there in our amazing brains. In Oxygen Yoga, the brain is the great control center, as it is for all other parts of life.

* * * OGA NOTE * * *

The concept of O2 and her flow through our beings, her on-going beneficial grace, and her effect on every move we make is much more broad, more profound, extensive and all-pervading than it may first appear. We can see it easily simply by looking at the skin of a long time smoker---the pallor, the wrinkling, the general, rapid aging of the skin is very obvious.

We use the deeply empowering stretching-out of our bodies with the yoga poses and their quieting effect on the unnecessary chatter in our thinking process. The use of breathing a healthy mix of air is to enhance our brains, and to treat our brains to a maximum intake of oxygen.

These practices have come down from the ancients—through the Vedas, the Taoists, and all the other wonderful centers of thought.

Originally controlled, full bellows use of our lungs inserted a fine mix of air by simply doing deep breathing practices. But those days are gone, so with pollution's smog soup, we have introduced added O_2 to bring us back to our full potential.

The original exercises worked their way down through the joint mind of human beings as we came together, moving toward harmony. The great truths are held sacred even now, and the versatility of the mind is one of its instruments we use for understanding those truths.

The body's fabulous capacity for multi-tasking and being versatile never capitulates from fear, never dissolves into a puddle, and never panics while seeking the imagined security of stasis. We may bog down in discursive thoughts but our beings always seek improved circumstances for their existence.

Oxygen Yoga is a miracle sprung forth from that never ending search of our minds. It just keeps plugging with its many tasks, doing thing as well as possible. The great news is that, as an extension, an aid to our brains, the oxygen can give them some real help.

Oxygen Yoga uses the inventions humans have devised and brought air to us in a clarified form, as is required for true, empowered breathing. Weighing less than three pounds, the brain is the main processor, the Central Processing Unit for human beings. As we all know, though compact and lightweight, it is an astonishing, sorting-out tool.

A NUMBER OF FACTORS ARE INVOLVED IN AGING

- Environmental degradation and the lack of a suitable mix of air is of course a major contributor to aging, especially in a time when medicine can cure us of so many ailments.
- The effects of our general disposition, a negative attitude, a defeating philosophy, continual strife, worrying so much that we feel stressed out. Research makes it look more and more as if the internal workings of our psyche are deeply related to rapid aging.

Firing up the circuitry of our body and mind, so that our connection with the universe opens further, can allow us to melt into the great vastness of being. As we move toward that enlightened being, the silence around us becomes counsel and we know the power of peace. We understand that our wonderful thinking machine is the center of our universe. Finally, we are sensing freedom, a meltdown of our protective shell that keeps us from being close to our environment.

That shell—not to be confused with the natural defense mechanisms that creatures use to nurture their existence in a world fraught with genuine threats like automobile collisions—can be relaxed.

Oga, with meditation and stretching of Yoga, can liberate us from the trap of too much thinking. A look at practicing Oxygen Yoga helps us with the understanding of our bodies, and with knowing them well and keeping in touch with them. It is not farfetched to see that the brain has a lot to do with keeping us youthful and invigorated. Getting a rein on the aging mechanisms gives Oga a special powerhouse quality.

In the end, it is all about aging with dignity, with strength, with gusto and a wonderful, positive view-point. These aspects of a life well-lived are all parts of reaching a higher level of consciousness. As we begin to work *with* our brain, rather than struggling with ourselves, we expand the intellect. Allowing ourselves peace of mind while learning to know when to give the body rest and when to exercise opens new vistas for the preservation of youthfulness.

As we develop self awareness through the use of oxygen, creating peace of mind with Oga, we open portals of thoughtfulness within ourselves.

Once the reader understands this booklet, she will move on automatically, by ordering a copy of the textbook, *Oxygen Yoga Pure & Simple* and searching down the classes in the Resources Guide. As the philosophy of Oga brings the practitioner closer into contact with all aspects of their beings, the basic knowledge of the peace that we already know begins to soothe us.

* * * OGA NOTE * * *

As civilization thickened and moved into the machine age, the urge to press forward with industrial pursuit, with the grasping for material accumulation overwhelmed the dignity of the ordinary person. We dropped the early forms of slavery, only to become indentured servants to the industrial revolution, and finally to our globalization by the corporate oligarchy. In the process numerical aging extended but not with full vitality—air polluting has inhibited vigor in each and every one of us. And, as slaves to wages and possessions, we tend to bypass the song of our hearts, which deadens our radiance.

The potent aid of Oxygen Yoga can actually help you develop new pathways throughout your brain. People enjoy predilections for various types of expression: music, words, dance, and the arts. Those who move best within the format of the arts, often look for ways of expressing their reaction to Oxygen Yoga. During a session, one may experience things that they have never thought before, never felt, and which they can't even describe.

The practice is based on learning to combine the concepts of age, time and creation and taking them all into the human psyche at once, then allowing the mind to emerge in it's totality. With Oga a person senses their work as an even more powerful self discovery process. The first step is always dropping our habit of clutching our thoughts tightly.

Although we appreciate and use oxygen as a supplement during yoga, the name Oxygen Yoga actually comes from a scientific study regarding the life flow in the brain which cannot continue without oxygen. The brain will stop. The oxygen also allows for the maximum mental experience. We cannot see an oxygen molecule, we can't even feel it, and we wouldn't even know we needed it until someone informed us.

Getting fully in touch with our human existence and the life forces requires our opening to the powers within, then learning to recognize the great forces of the universe by learning to feel into ourselves, by seeing ourselves as blank slates ready to be written upon with new information— much the same as children do naturally. As one begins to fully comprehend what a masterful creation the human brain is, gets familiar with its full capabilities, appreciation of one's own self develops. Taking care of this life we are given takes on new importance.

By the realization of our true selves, our inherent value, and seeing the abundance of life on this earth, one can essentially prevent premature aging. There are many unknowns in the human brain, and because the discovery of one's full potential is so rich, we must build a sound foundation. Science is not separate and apart from us. We are science. We are each finely tuned, highly orchestrated and complex creations designed to fulfill our purpose on this earth.

Think of the oxygen around you, giving your brain what it requires to remain healthy and functional. Inhale deeply. Imagine the feeling of a proper mix of air flooding every nook and cranny of your being. Allow your mind to use your thoughts to create peaceful, calming effects upon the body. Breathing helps make the calm all pervading. Endorphins will flow and may join other natural compounds that can even lighten the load of aches and pain.

With the adoption of Oga into your daily life, you will begin to eliminate stress from your mind by recognizing that you have been placed on this earth for a purpose and that you are a very special creation. Your sense of intent will allow you to accept your native gifts and open the doors for giving them to the world around you.

As you move into the totality of Oga, *Oxygen Yoga Pure & Simple,* your innate attention to the beauty of the natural environment, to a flower and its intricacies, to the smiles of friends, will open themselves up to you more and more. You will gaze into the heavens and admire the beauty of the clouds and the blueness of the sky. Let your mind drift and open up to the wonders of the universe and all it has to offer. The mind and it's amazing ride on the oxygen in our blood governs our perception, our ability to be aware of our senses in so many ways—it is our fabulous guide, and we can learn to rest in the eclipse of it, to get grounded, and fully centered and short circuit many of the hardships that a modern life hurls our way.

CHAPTER 3

POLLUTION AND THE AIR WE BREATHE

Breathing and oxygen combine to form a marvel, one of those great treasures of the universe: the sun shining upon green leaves and producing oxygen; the rain giving life to a seed; the gravity keeping us put; our own discovery of deep-healing environments.

Throughout the breathtaking expanse of interstellar space, we find fabulous gases in all their wonderful skirts and swirls, moving and dancing with energy. The heat and winds of other gasses carry them up and roll them around and around, pushing them into all their varied forms. The gases perform miracles in their abundance and their racing madness—gases working in conjunction in a waltz with all living creatures.

* * * OGA NOTE * * *

Everything on this earth operates in an orderly manner, a coming together; all has been designed that way. The entities of the coming together prefer to be neutral together—or as close to neutral as possible.

The oxygen molecule is a perfect example. It prefers to exist as O2, rather than lingering as a plain old O. If they are not conjoined, they look for a mate, much like ourselves, seeking relationships with one another and with God, a place to bond. It is why cells reproduce—the energy in them dissipates and the radicals figure out who they are and they are expelled. Otherwise, there would not be any room for new cells. Everything has a purpose. Everyone has a purpose.

Our brains create our universe, serve as the mega-center for what we know as our lives and they are very dependent on the amount of O_2 available in the blood. Oxygen meanders through our bodies in our rich, iron laden, chemically charged blood cells and brings her zing to every fiber of our being. From the moment of conception—and even well before—we need oxygen. We can only exist for a few minutes without a robust, roiling supply of O_2 providing her spark to our brains. And it must be a never-ending, twenty percent charge of her that is with us all through our lives. With a pure, clean, supply of Oxygen, we human beings came to the zenith of survival that we now enjoy.

She is a molecule formed by a simple grouping of atoms. For now, let's think of oxygen taking shape as a small circle, so small that you cannot see it. In fact, O_2 is a lot smaller than a cell. The molecule is held together like a magnet otherwise, it would fall apart. The outer electrons circle the nucleus like planets around the sun.

NOTHING IN ANY OXYGEN YOGA PROCRAM SHOULD CAUSE PAIN

- Oga is simply about providing conditions for regaining the natural supply of Oxygen for which human beings are designed
- There should never be pain involved with your practice
- This applies to everyone.
- All certified Oga teachers should teach the same principles.
- If you are in pain, you must consult with your instructor immediately.

- Be sure to read the Oxygen Yoga Pure & Simple textbook with great care and stay fully in tune with your classes and instructors.

The atomic forces hold everything in place. As we mentioned, oxygen molecules do not like to face existence alone, so they are always looking for a companion. Together, they feel much more stable and complete, just like us human beings. This is their calling. It is etched in the flow of the universe, and like so many of Mother Nature's miracles, the coming together of these molecules, their unrelenting drive to bond, provides life for us and many other creatures.

Oxygen is clear. You cannot see it, not even under a microscope. And, you cannot feel it, yet it surrounds our bodies all the time. It floats, moves and bounces on us and around us in constant motion continuously.

Though we cannot see it, can't separate it from the other gases around our bodies, don't even realize that it is always with us, oxygen is very real and, one-and-all, we have an extremely intimate relationship with it. Oxygen has been on this earth since the beginning of time as we know it.

As humans we only assemble things. We really don't create or invent anything. Everything that human beings put together comes from this earth, which was provided for us, already existing. Even vehicles that we design for space travel are composed from metals, ceramics and composites found in the earth.

* * * OGA NOTE * * *

As we have noted, Oxygen can sometimes provide the effect of oxidation, which is the chemical reaction that creates rust in metals. Imagine this happening to your skin. The skin's protective shield is broken down and it is put directly in a horrid path of exposure. The epidermis turns red, blisters, causes pain and may even turn into cancer. Pain is one of the fabulous warning signs with which we are blessed. But, we are not always that swift at heeding the alarms. The oldest truths, the obvious thoughts, are often the wisest, and we take them for granted so easily. Not only are they wise, but also written at face value— if something causes one pain, it should clearly be avoided.

When we are breathing air that is deeply polluted as we do for most of our lives, all of our receptors and mental states are thrown off balance. Thinking becomes

erratic rather than smooth and stable. Our natural, genetic concern for safety within our environment is thrown askew and paranoia sets in to our every fiber.

When we operate from a base of fear, we attempt to convince ourselves how superior, how magnificent we are. We fog over our clarity—the fright causes us to move into speed and aggression. We forget to relax with the wonderful creatures we are. It is a vast tragedy that insecurity triggers us to reeling around in these bouts of trying to convince ourselves that we are better than others, of playing "prove-it."

As humans we are good gathers, collectors, linear thinkers and assemblers. However, if the walls of our linear constructs don't line up, many of our species move into attack mode. The Oxygen Yoga program, using the basic tool of meditation and the natural expansion of mind that comes with the Oga practice can rein in our egos to their natural, healthy state.

All creatures have very purposeful lives. There are actually organisms that can exist without O_2. The reason that these organisms, free of the need for oxygen, have been preserved is that they were located in places not exposed to the environment. Their very existence illustrates yet another miraculous part of our ecosystem. In the great flow of the universe, there is never a thought that we evolved from these beings and later decided to develop lungs just to breathe oxygen. The whole circle of life is much grander than fear-based, human, reactionary thoughts can grasp.

Humans require a steady stream of O_2, an average of a cup or so per minute. Of that supply, twenty percent or so goes to the brain—which is only a couple percent of the entire body's mass. Unless we are in the Himalaya or kayaking the Bering Straight, we use between two and three thousand gallons a day. Some of the questions we may have about the effect of the lack of oxygen on our brain and bodies can be answered very simply just by looking at the changes we go through during exercise and when we are still. With the pollution of the skies effecting the makeup of the ambient air, one begins to see how difficult the conditions become for our bodies. Exercising in bad air can actually cause harm.

* * * OGA NOTE * * *

With the practice, the spiral toward the end of our life here on this earth becomes clearer to the practitioner. The awareness brings life into focus and it becomes even more precious.

One begins to know that the more often the twenty percent balance of oxygen is present in our environments, the more fulfilling each year becomes. We begin to understand that there will always be bumps in the road. We know that they will be there for us every single day of our lives. We learn to become one with frightening thoughts like aging and learn to know that it is just another verse in the song of our hearts. As we master the process of working with life, we feel and look younger and age is overshadowed by radiance.

With bad air, changes in skin color are obvious, as is the heaviness of breathing. As we utilize our muscles, we feel our strength increase. If we have a decent mix of O_2, a sense of mastery and power comes over us as we feel our chests swell and we experience an increase in visceral awareness of our local environs. Oxygen provides energy to every one of our cells of perception.

When the oxygen is adequate, the metabolism is said to be aerobic. When the demand for energy is lowered, a less efficient form of breathing known as anaerobic metabolism is engaged. As one begins to exercise, the anaerobic pathways provide for the initial boost of ATP—adenosine triphosphate—while the body shifts into gear to increase supplying oxygen to the cells. Food energy is released via ATP.

This increase leads to faster breathing and heart rates. The more oxygen is transported to the exercising cells, the more the aerobic pathways pick up the slack. The anaerobic part tapers off. In Oga, one works with the Yoga poses smoothly but with a strong command of the musculature. They require a good deal of draw on one's energy supply, which in turn, requires that the precious gas is brought into our bodies abundantly.

However, this entire process is derailed by the shortage of O_2 in the ambient air we breathe. As we all know, our bodies survive for weeks without food and days without water but only a few minutes without oxygen. O_2 is everywhere on earth. However, we have developed Oga due to the fact that we simply do not have the natural composition of clean, pure air with oxygen as 21% of the gases that make up our breath supply.

Once you pick up your copy of *Oxygen Yoga Pure & Simple* and begin a regular practice you will begin to counteract the global pollution and the air we breathe. If your workout is only a few times a week, imagine how overjoyed your body will be to able to put the miracle of O_2 to full use.

CHAPTER 4

LETTING THE BODY QUIET THE MIND

One of the most fabulous qualities of our human design is the seamless integration of the entire, conscious entity that we call ourselves. And, equally stunning is the spot-on meld of our interior—through our fibrous skin—to our great conjunction with the entire universe.

The elegance of Oxygen Yoga can be seen over and over again, and one of the most striking visions of the power of the Oga process is the natural sheen we develop that includes the entirety of our beings. That shine is not simply limited to the results of stretching of musculature, which does work wonders for the body. Oga goes farther; the movements combined with O_2 spread over the entire body. And then, as the mind lets go, drops the endless roar of interior prattle, the body is effected thoroughly.

As the novitiate winds along the way, the knowledge that during the physical movements, while one is paying attention to a pose, holding it, and practicing awareness—a good deal more than simple stretching transpires. And, during the meditation, it becomes more and more obvious that one contemplates the being as a very special creation, right along side the beautiful and giving earth and the magnificence of simply being alive.

This profound work puts one thoroughly in touch with the universe in a literal way; we can feel our expansiveness. To get a taste of the opening that you will begin to experience, take some time, fifteen minutes or so, and work with this little exercise. Relax, do not rush, breath deeply, close the eyes and imagine a luxuriant, white tropical flower, focus on the soft dark blue sky behind, and in the background, feel green water softly rippling in the wind. Take your time and allow your senses to have command.

Experience the entire episode as timelessness. This is an Oxygen Yoga teaching. You will resound immediately to the great fullness your experience, to the beauty and realize that it is a mind-body experience. It is the closest we can come to "stopping the clock" aside from death. There are many techniques such as meditation, visualization, color therapy, relaxation, imagery, hypnosis, and more, which can lead to physiological healing by quieting the mind. But the use of a healthy supply of O_2 is what makes this work unique. Did the fantasy make you smile? What were your authentic, automatic reactions? It presents a small taste of Oxygen Yoga.

After you have begun your practice of Oga, looking at yourself, feeling into the new awareness that yoga and meditation brings, it will become straightforward for you to gain an idea of how the mind-body connection works. The yoga movements and conscious breathing begin to quiet the mad racing of mind because they require singular attention. Any form of meditation will further your ability to keep from being grabbed up in the mind's horrid, internal, series of diatribes that pull one away from simple enjoyment of the present moment—from happiness.

In *Oxygen Yoga Pure & Simple*, we move into more detail, guide you into a close look at the brain and its pathways, which lead to every organ of our body. You will learn to feel the mind-body connection just by waking up in the morning.

With the new supply of oxygen along with the quieting of your mind, you will begin to feel refreshed and revitalized most of the time, and when you don't, it will be due to some substance that you have ingested, to stress, or it will have arisen from illness.

* * * OGA NOTE * * *

Think of yourself as existing in the present, in a time warp, a place where time does not exist, where the ever changing moment has become ordinary. Now, allow yourself to NOT- FEEL your body, to feel weightless. Let the attention rest at one point on your forehead between you eyebrows. This is the only part you can feel—like a burning, hot sensation, a volcano. Now, make it feel cooler like a polar ice cap. Breathe slow and deep. After practicing enough, your brain will start to cleanse itself, images will begin to appear like a dream, and you will begin to notice what you have never seen before. Thoughts that have never ever arisen will surface. Do not hurry. Don't panic. Allow yourself to experience the entire episode as timelessness.

You will not only feel the enhancements of Oga resonate fully with the information in *Oxygen Yoga Pure & Simple*, but all of your activity, your resting time, your erratic life will feel markedly more rich and full.

Many complaints that you have endured for years are apt to begin to slip away. Your sleep and dream-state can become very elegant. Sleep and feeling rested are another of the great miracles, a time when we automatically stop the world and slip into the vast dreamscape to chill out and mend.

The study of sleep and disorders related to the nation's endemic lack of deep, rich sleep are a whole science unto themselves. Even the proponents of legal drugs and the full spectrum of so-called, modern, medical science are exploring the effects of ancient healing practices like meditation. Researchers conduct continual studies of how external events produce physiological change in the body due to how we deal with the events.

The expansive classification which is a variety of disorders being explored in this work, are labeled psychosomatic. The term is commonly misunderstood—a basic assumption that the patient has fantasized their complaints often prevails. The working premise then becomes— these phenomenons are merely figments of the imagination and therefore, are of no importance.

But that supposition is not the case at all. By disregarding a person's complaints, a great wall of denial is mortared into place. Our pain and suffering are very real, of true, profound substance no matter whether manifested from blunt force trauma in an automobile accident, resultant of the gnawing of voices from family trauma that torment us solely from within the psyche.

One of the most substantial effects of the practice of Oxygen Therapy is the way in which our minds quiet down; the amazing fact that many fears, upon coming into focus, are exposed as chimeras of pointless worrying ourselves; and simply being released from dwelling on that anguish can allow it to evaporate with our exhales of unneeded gases from our lungs. Through the practice of Oga, many pains may simply fade because the practitioner's being is growing more and more at ease with itself. Your practice of Oxygen Yoga should never cause pain—if it appears to be causing you discomfort, confide with your teacher immediately

PSYCHOSOMATIC DOES NOT MEAN THAT THE AILMENTS DO NOT EXIST

- Psycho-physiological skin disorders such as neurodermatitis (inflammation) and hyperhydrosis.
- Respiratory disorders such as bronchial asthma and hyperventilation.

- Gastrointestinal disorders: peptic ulcers, chronic gastritis, ulcerative or mucous colitis, constipation, and heartburn.
- Cardiovascular disorders such as tachycardia (heart racing), hypertension, and migraine headache.
- Genitourinary disorders such as disturbances in menstruation and urination, dyspareunia (painful sexual intercourse), and impotence.
- Musculoskeletal disorders like backaches, muscle cramps, and tension headaches.
- If you feel these or any symptoms, be sure to consult with your Doctor, to read the *Oxygen Yoga Pure & Simple textbook* and to consult with your instructor. Oga is not a practice of medicine. If symptoms arrive or disappear, pay close attention with great care and stay fully in tune with your physicians, classes and instructors.

Some of these disorders will be familiar to most readers, and the fact that they can drop by the wayside with the Oga practice will be a powerful insight. This realization will paint a graphic picture of the great power of the mind-body connection. The significant understanding that you may come to with these syndromes, could be that psychosomatic conditions aggravated by pollution of the natural environment, are a serious threat. They are the principal force of the disorders.

Pain is not the insignificant imaginings of the sufferer; and obviously, those listed are not direct responses to outside influences like blunt-trauma, lacerations, or bacterial invasions. The body produces pain as a result of conditions in the environment that it perceives as disruptive for its healthy functioning. Naturally, the effects are the same as with any illness. A person can die from "psychologically produced" high blood pressure exactly as if the pressure came from any cause. The mind can produce debilitating physiological change, but can it actually heal us?

In many research projects, a placebo or pharmacologically inert substance has been introduced to the study, and the involved persons have associated the placebo with beneficial physiological change due to the person's belief that the substance would work. These instances are not new, medical science has been aware of this connection for quite some time, especially in the field of pain relief. Specifically, a placebo administered as a drug that would aid relief has exactly that effect.

The question then becomes—how much of our wellness is produced by our relationship to ourselves, to a positive outlook, to a strong, stretched-out body. And the thought grows thicker if we see the possibility in re-introducing the twenty-odd percent of O_2 into our air stream? The great well of calm that resides there within, just sitting there in the person's being, waiting for the patient to use in relieving pain somehow activates from the faith invested in a placebo.

If a simple suggestion is full of such potential, it is easy to imagine the power of Oga. And with Oxygen Yoga at work, the body's natural pain suppression systems cause other, natural forces such as the release of beta-endorphins to launch. Given that the mind can influence physiological processes in the body, both for good and ill, the question becomes: do the standard, commonly mental, non-medical healing strategies somehow tap into whatever mind-body relationship is responsible for producing positive physiological change? In other words, do these common techniques from outside the medical industry heal the body? Research indicates that some of the non-medical techniques are associated with beneficial physiological change.

There is research that supports an association between imagination and physiological processes.

Studies have found that individuals who imagine an event often undergo the bodily changes associated with actual participation in it and are prone to enjoy maximum benefits from the activity, if the image is positive.

During this type of imagery session one is presented with an optimal time for incorporating relaxing, stretching exercises and oxygen for the lungs into the process. The Oga practice is used to promote healing, to cleanse and to detoxify the system. This results in full optimization of the brain and body. The techniques for the poses work well with O_2 as strong aids to anti-aging. We invite you to join us and experience this deep sense of well being for yourself.

CHAPTER 5

OXYGENIZED YOGA CHANGES BEING ALIVE

The origins of Oxygen Yoga reach back into the past, into an ancient and very deep pool of knowledge. Since the beginnings of the Vedic Traditions in India thousands of years ago the postures of Yoga have been developing. Humans allowed the voices of the heavens to speak through them; the great insight of the Yoginis and Yogins began to arise as teachings. From the beginnings of the Vedas in India, the power of breath has been known as sacred.

The great truths from those ancient times came to be known in many places as well as with the Indian Masters: Tibetan Yoga, the movements of the Toltec, the Taoist full breath work.

The Greeks used the term pneuma and in today's English we still use derivative words like pneumatic. Plato himself worked with the breath—the psyche being a combination of spirit and being alive and the psyche's air and the fire of it were in every fiber of our tissue. In this Classical Greek thinking, not only did humans enjoy this aliveness of air circulation, all things did.

Chi, mana, Orinda, Od, sugs, prana, pneuma: oxygen has been one of our most deeply understood symbols and it always refers to the force that flows through us as life by whatever set of terms the ancients expressed the great, deep power of our oneness with the universe. And always, throughout these powerful teachings, the teachers eulogize the profound effects of deep breathing, the fact that a continued practice changes being alive.

Being close to the heavens, unadulterated by smog and modern lights, the originators of thorough stretching felt the mysteries with great vibrance, knew them in their heartbeat, in the very depths of their souls. From this early wealth of experience, so close to the elements, to the breathing of heaven, the natural forms of Yoga arose.

As deep and simple as the luminous water at the bottom of an open, twenty foot well, as powerful and overwhelming as the great Himalaya, the in and out, the dance of oxygen is vast, and always at play.

Those early human conversations with the universe still reflect the vastness, the inborn understanding that we all share. And we still use them in Oxygen Yoga. However, in those early millennia, the natural environment had not been pillaged monumentally—fresh air was abundant.

* * * OGA NOTE * * *

If we learn the fiery power of the knowledge that has been handed down to us with care, we can use the breath as we have all great tools. As we use the power of the common hammer to construct the most basic elements of a built-environment, we can get in touch with our breath to feel the strength of mind as it melts into union with the universe.

However, we must remember to work in a skilful manner or we can injure ourselves. In the same way, Yoga poses require exertion and we must heed the depth of breathing so it assists rather than hinders us. We must be very aware the intake can even become harmful as busy lungs take in larger doses of toxins than passive lungs do.

One of the beauties of Oga is that your teacher will introduce Pure O2 into the mix of ambient air. Infusing the body with it is one of the reasons that Oxygen Yoga brings so much of the awareness of mystery and in-depth understanding to the practitioners.

Discovery by the elders led to the deep breathing required for the sometimes strenuous movements of Hatha Yoga. There was no need to incorporate the intake of O_2. The Masters passed the teachings on to the gentry, taught them to pull into the being on the in-breath, to learn release and out-giving with the exhalation—to flow into the steady pool of being.

Working with teachers of true understanding, with a teaching like Oxygen Yoga that clearly overwhelms ego, the practitioner comes alive taking in a deep, profoundly healing and enervating dose of oxygen in its natural state.

Since those early periods of human life, we have pushed on and on with our curious brains, producing the machinations of the heavy pollution of this age. And with that same brilliance of our minds, we can open to our voices as the ancients did. Collectively we can lead the corporations and the politicians away from our current destructive behavior, and start bringing all of the components to work for our enjoined spirit. We can produce fine work like organic farms, solar energy, and green buildings. If we learn the fiery power of the breath-knowledge handed down to us with care for many centuries, we can use our breathing as we have all great aids.

Hatha Yoga is the most widespread form, the one most of us have heard of, and have practiced. Though it is the most well known, there are other forms of yoga. Raja Yoga is a scientific path that defines the teachings with great care. In the Raja, our human behavior is broken into limbs, or parts.

THE Eight LIMBSOF THE ROYAL ROAD ARE

- Yama - The rules of social behavior
- Niyama - The rules of personal behavior
- Asana - Which means seat or pose?
- Pranayama - The mastering of our life force through our breath
- Pratyahara - Directing the senses inward via meditation
- Dharana - The mastery of attention and intention.
- Dhyana - Developing the witnessing of awareness.

- Samadhi - Uniting with the spirit.

Hatha Yoga is the great tool for knowing the wealth of our bodies and it develops the practice from the use of the limbs: The three limbs are asana, pranayana, and pratyahara.

When we break Hatha into syllables and delve into the history of the Vedic tradition and Sanskrit a bit, we find that the two syllables represent the Sun—Ha, and the Moon—Tha. With this snippet of knowledge it is simple enough to see why many refer to Hatha Yoga as the form that finds the union of our beings through the understanding found in opposites.

These sets practiced when engaging in Hatha Yoga give it distinctness, a standing on its own as the more forceful yoga because it requires the most physical exercises of all the form of yoga. Through a combination of proper breathing, meditation and physically challenging poses, practitioners can achieve balanced, all-around development of human potential while promoting health and well being.

As pointed out in the list above, the asanas or the core physical teachings are very important in Yoga. And, central to the asana practice is the mastery of breathing in order to assume the often complex poses that are required of the practitioner.

In addition, the Sanatan Society—an international group that provides profound information about the culture of India—states that "If one can master breath, then the mastery of the mind is within reach. Through breathing exercises the flow of prana or vital life force through the body is regulated." This significant mastery of one's being is absolutely essential for long-term, in-depth fulfillment of the further steps one climbs in Hatha Yoga.

The practice brings balance to the two hemispheres of the brain—and, at last, springing the practitioner into the ability of activating what is known as Kundalini energy. The great and infinitely powerful medium of the Kundalini is considered to be an energy waiting to be awakened that will move through our being to create an optimal energized life. Through the practice of asana, pranayama and pratyahara (hatha) people can awaken the life force within and connect with the divine consciousness.

Why Practice Yoga in the first place? Why not just buy a tank of O2 and benefit from a proper mix of air? In order to lead a long and healthy lifestyle, there are many things a person must do. At the very top of that list is engaging in physical activity. All deep-thinking people since the beginning of human thought have recognized that using our bodies is one of the most essential elements in maintaining a healthy state of being.

* * * OGA NOTE * * *

Maharishi Patangali—one of the great sages from India—brought depth and substance to modern yoga practices. He pinned down, and clearly defined the eight aspects of living one works with on the journey to our connection with our higher self. The Mahrishi strengthened yoga as one of the great Paths for uniting with the highest consciousness of the universe. His remarkable efforts in bringing about the great spiritual investigations of the various teachers together, has been a magnificent contribution to all of us who have come since. As you pursue Oga, and by reading the *Oxygen Yoga Pure & Simple,* **textbook you will begin to take in ample O$_2$ while working with your teacher. You will feel the tradition of clarity that we are blessed with from the ancients.**

Oxygen Yoga is a full system of physical, mental and spiritual exercises that encompasses the whole being. There are many benefits of the practice.

Muscles and bones will gain strength for better balance and more power. Stretching of the muscles and joints will allow for a more limber body. In addition, the cardiovascular and respiratory systems will be worked to help build stamina. Performing yoga poses while practicing conscious breathing will enable one to become more centered. Being centered means that the silly pursuits of inflated ego move into the background and calming thoughts move into the foreground of the psyche. The psyche will then be allowed to participate fully in the wealth of experience that is present wherever we may be during our lives.

CHAPTER 6

THE FIRST STEP BEGINS NOW

Our Spiritual Journey, the Path, the Way, the passage of our spirits through our lifetime is found referenced in sacred texts around the globe and referenced in many ways. This often mentioned Path; the great Journey of the spiritual seeker is the route to enlightenment that rests in all hearts.

It is easy enough to see that providing a sweeping flush of our being with a well balanced mix of oxygen, which provides the very breath of life herself, is extremely important. Now, more than ever—with our little planet gone toxic from global corporate negligence—keeping close watch over our breath is absolutely imperative.

As one begins to realize what a boost the intake of our primary survival need in its healthy form can give to our being, it is easy to see that with a basic grasp of Oxygen Yoga technique, your astounding journey can begin. You do not need to sit around for years, trying to build up credentials to become an enlightened person.

With *Oxygen Yoga Pure & Simple*, you simply follow the instructions, and pay careful attention to the poses in the accompanying photographs. Your teacher will help you understand what is taking place. Your fellow practitioners will help you explore the depth of the knowledge.

Here, in the handbook, we will take an introductory look at the postures themselves to help you see what we are doing. The following are several different Yoga poses that will later become a part of your own practice.

As you move farther into the work you will require the carefully prepared images displayed in *Oxygen Yoga Pure & Simple* to help you understand what you are doing and to be able to focus on your positioning. Working with your teacher, you will require an O_2 headset and you will take time to get comfortable with it before beginning to exercise.

Your focus in Oga will be the upper body, but you will also balance and ground yourself throughout the lower energy centers. In the feet, legs, hips and base of spine we harness the earth's energy and continue moving energy upward into the pelvis and then tap into our core energy source.

As you enter the core or solar plexus area you can engage the power that already lives within us. The energy radiates up into The Heart Center and connects with our breath. Then it continues moving upward into the throat area, which is the communication center. Next, on the upward trail, it moves to the forehead which is The Third Eye Center. This is where we connect with our higher self, our spirit.

From the Third Eye allow your prana to expand further up into the crown area, which is the top of your head. Naturally, the crown is the highest point of connection, with the most elevated energy, we connect there with our universal source—the consciousness from which everything originated. With the breath and meditation the precise physical movements, or asana, are also required. All of our efforts in the Oxygen Yoga are extremely important.

As you work with the Oxygen Yoga poses, you must also practice awareness, paying keen attention to the eight primary centers: Root, Sacral, Solar Plexus, Heart, Throat, Third Eye, Crown and the Aura of energy that surrounds your being, which can be considered the eighth center.

THE EIGHT ENERGY CENTERS

- Root
- Sacral
- Solar Plexus
- Heart
- Throat
- Third Eye
- Crown
- The Aura

Because the energy centers radiate how we are feeling, it is essential that we learn to tame our fluctuating thoughts by allowing them to become still—neither fighting to push them away or grasping to hold on to our moods.

Oxygen Yoga is a fabulous tool for working with energy centers, for bringing them into balance. You will see in the following pages how all the above information comes together to assist you in your journey. Embrace the essence of each of the centers as you practice your first Oxygen Yoga session. From the core down is your power, from the heart up is light and energy generating upward toward the sun. The eighth Chakra is the protective energy center around you; grow it further outward, starting from within and radiating to the world. Your increasing health and wholeness will expand with your own liberation from the bindings of ego. Your expanded radiance will benefit others with great Love. Let your being radiate peace and harmony as it relearns its native ability to shine. This greatest of all journeys begins as you step onto The Path, moving toward the ultimate goal of Enlightenment. It is our connection with the Divine.

THE POSES

1. Breathe Pose – When you move into *Oxygen Yoga Pure & Simple* and begin work with your teacher, you will put on your head set and use oxygen. For now, lay on your back with your right hand on your chest area. Put your left hand on your belly area. Elbows should be resting on the floor. Exhale through your mouth creating a "haaaaah" sound to encourage awareness of your breath. Inhale through your nose inflating your lower belly first; continue the breath slowly upward to the chest. Continue breathing slower and slower in and out through the nose. Each breath begins from the low belly in or out. This is called "belly" or diaphragmic breathing. Each breath should become

slower and longer. At some point, as you breathe and relax, you will begin to feel like your breath is breathing you. Of course, all will be enhanced with oxygen, and, remember that one should work with an instructor to avoid injury. Exhaling is always an opportunity to release any stress you may have. Continue for at least 5-10 minutes and feel the peace within.

2.   Bridge Pose – bend your knees with your feet on the floor. Your feet and knees should be spread to hip width. Put your heels under the knees. Lift the hips off the floor and place your arms under your back. Move shoulder blades in towards each other. Interlace hands with palms facing each other. Lift the chest as well as hips. Breathe slow, deep and big. Practice three or more sets of breaths.

3.   Oxygen Awakening Pose – from Bridge Pose, move arms to your sides and relax your spine onto the ground one vertebrae at a time. Bend your knees up into the chest and roll onto your side. Sit up and cross your legs. Inhale while lifting both arms above your head to generate energy

flowing up from your grounding seat, up through the head. Be fully aware of uplifting the lower energies awaking the heart center. Expand your ribs and chest upward, stretching the spine. Exhale while reaching both arms out to the side, away from each other, opening your front shoulders. Bring your arms behind you and press the hands gently into the floor. Inhale as you open the chest and ribs upward and forward, expanding into the breast bone. Gently focus your breathing lightly, slowly, and deeply into awakening your lungs. Let go of your neck and shoulders as your shoulder blades reach toward each other in your upper back. Breathe 3 sets of breaths or more while in the position.

4. Seated Side Stretch Pose – continue from The Oxygen Awakening Pose, inhale as you float both arms out to the side, then, while they are above the head, reaching upward fully. Stretch your spine. As you exhale, bring your left arm down directly to the left side, hand on the floor. Raise your right arm even higher, up to the sun and then exhale opening the right

rib cage as you stretch over to the left. Breathe deeply and steadily for three or more sets. Keep your neck and shoulders relaxed and melting downward. As you exhale, bring both arms down beside you, then inhale the arms up again, and then change sides.

5. Cow Tilt Pose – move on to your hands and knees. Put hands directly under shoulders while knees are placed under hips. Inhale, lifting your chin upward and exhale with your back down through your belly like a saddle. Look upward with eyes. Shoulders should be pressing firmly down into the hands keeping arms straight. The inner elbows should be facing each other. Stretch into the abdominals, chest and neck. Gently lift the buttocks upward. Complete three sets of breaths.

6. Cat Pose – exhale from the Cow Pose. Press navel into spine as if hollowing out the belly area. Arch back up to the sky with head down and chin tucked into the chest. Shoulders must remain strong, moving through arms and into hands.

Complete three sets of breathes while arched here.

7. Open Lung Mountain Pose – from Cat Pose, slowly come to standing into the Open Lung Mountain Pose. Bring legs forward, one at a time and place feet under chest on the floor. Lift up to a standing position pressing your feet firmly into the ground. Rest your arms to your sides. Inhale as arms open outward and then float them up above the shoulders. Energize the fingers. Align shoulders, hips and feet making sure all four corners of feet are evenly weighted and placed. Feel the power, strength and stability from the earth move into your feet; up into your legs through the abdominals and all the energizing up through your core center. As you strengthen downward from the core simultaneously energize upward as well. Breathe slowly, taking in big, deep breaths. Feel your body's alignment and balance. Open the heart upward and outward. Expand into the space around you. Find your body's alignment. This Pose creates your connection with

the earth and is your basic pose for all others.

8. Standing Back Bend – Back Bend from Open Lung Mountain Pose, inhale moving arms above head, thumbs together lifting the chest and ribs up to the sky. Exhale while moving your head and arms and shoulders backward. Inhaling while here will bring you further upward. Each exhale gently brings you deeper into your backbend. Open the heart center, chest, lungs upward. Strengthen your energy down into feet and thighs from the core to the earth. Breathe slowly, taking in long, deep breaths. Complete three sets or more. Mid and lower body are powerful and grounding. The upper body is light, long and energized upward from the heart center. The stronger your lower body is pressing downward, the safer and easier it is to comfortably go into your backbend.

9. Brain Stimulating Standing Forward Bend Pose – From backward bend; exhale and dive forward slowly. Lead the dive with the chest while reaching arms out to

the side. Next, grasp hands together behind your back and gently straighten arms as far back as possible. It is alright to bend your knees and elbows if needed. Continue by folding down from hips, not the waist. Allow your head to gently relax as your chin tucks into chest lightly. This will create a light stretch in your neck. Take in a long, deep breath. Stand evenly on each foot, applying slightly more weight in the front big toe and balls of your feet. It is important to remember not to lean too much into your heels. Again, you may bend your knees to insure proper form, but make sure to keep a relaxed lower back.

10. Warrior One Pose – inhale up slowly from Standing Forward Bend Pose to a full standing position using the strength of your feet, legs and core. Once erect, bring the right leg straight back behind you and bend the front, left leg. The right foot should be at a 45 degree angle with toes facing slightly forward. Back heel should be touching the ground. Inhale and raise arms above your head, palms facing each other. Exhale slowly while strengthening your core and tap into

your inner power. Energize this power down through the thighs and into the feet. Feel the energy force from the earth exchanging with your inner power. Make sure your weight is equally distributed to both feet and legs while the torso is centered over the hips. Now, press your right hip forward to square your hips in front of you. Slide your shoulders down your back. Stretch up through your waist into your energized hands. Let each inhale lift the torso higher to create a long, strong stretch. Feel the energy moving through your body. Power through this pose, like a warrior, the best you can without straining or forcing anything. Allow your ujayii breath to assist you at all times. The breath is our way of connecting the body and mind. Finish and relax yours arms down to yours sides. Repeat on the opposite side. Switch legs and inhale arms up and over your head. Repeat the same steps on the opposite side. Make sure to complete three sets of breath on each side.

11.   High Pyramid Pose – from Warrior One Pose, exhale while moving your arms

down by your side and straighten front leg. Maintain the same foot placement as in Warrior One Pose. Inhale while opening your arms out to the sides and stretch into your front shoulders. Bring your arms behind your back and place your hands in the small of your back. Inhale into the heart center, upward to the sky. Expand your breathing to your breastbone. Relax your head gently backwards releasing your neck as well. Breathe slowly and deeply through the heart up to the heavens. Feel the energy. Lengthen your spine in front and back upward during each inhale. Exhale power out from your core down through your legs into the foundation of your feet. Feel the vibration from the earth, up, into your being and on up through your heart. When you feel the need to move to the other side after about three sets of breaths, then exhale. Exhale as you move the legs together standing in neutral Tadasana or Mountain Pose and switch to the other side to repeat high pyramid. Three sets of breaths or more should be practiced in this pose.

12. Downward Facing Dog Pose – from High Pyramid, lengthen torso upward bending the knees fold forward from hips bringing hands into the ground moving into an upside down "v" shape. The feet are as flat into the ground as possible, heels reaching for the earth. Elevate the "sit bones," reaching for the sky at the same time. Straighten your legs as much as comfortably possible. Press the floor away with your front palms lift the hips upward and press the heels down. As you press your navel into your spine, expand your rib cage outward. Keep a nice straight back do not curve into the spine. Move the shoulder blades away from each other and downward away from neck. Your hands should not be directly under your shoulders but far out in front of them. Inner elbows should face each other.

13. Cobra Pose – from downward dog move onto hands and knees, then straighten body forward onto the belly. Lift your chest and mid torso forward and upward by pressing into hands and arms. Move the shoulder blades down the back, gently pressing your pelvis into the floor. Stretch

your belly forward and upward through the chest with each inhale lifting the heart center and exhaling the hips back and down along with the shoulders. The legs are heavy with the feet into the ground. Three sets of breaths more or less should be practiced.

14. Seal Pose – sit back out of Cobra Pose. Bring hips back toward feet and sit as close to feet as comfortable. For knee issues, place a rolled up towel behind the knees for comfort. Relax the torso into the thighs. If possible, rest the forehead into the ground or use a folded towel or Yoga block on which to rest the forehead. Gently stretch the arms out to the front then rest the elbows onto the floor. Once in this position, your body should feel relaxed and loose. Think only about your breathing and feel your body moving, expanding and releasing as you inhale and exhale. Release your muscles, head, neck and shoulders. Let go of your hips, thighs and arms. You may move your arms backward resting them onto the floor with hands relaxing by the feet as well.

15. Crescent Moon Pose -- sit up slowly from seal pose, then onto hands and knees. Move the right leg forward and bend the right knee. Right foot should be directly under the right knee, comfortable, flat, with sole on the floor. The left leg should straighten as far and straight back as possible with the top of the left foot in the ground. Inhale as you lengthen your torso up toward the sky, making sure to open the heart center and breast bone. Exhale while moving the shoulders, head and arms backward behind you creating a beautiful arch with your back. Keep your hips as square as possible. Engage the base of the spine and pelvic muscles up into your spine and core to assist you in lifting upward. Remain grounded throughout the lower body and uplifted from the heart to the head. Breathe slowly and deeply. Enjoy the expansion. Perform three or more sets of breaths. Move from here into standing forward bend, before moving onto other side of crescent moon.

16. Water Fall Forward Bend Pose – move out of Crescent Moon by folding forward onto hands and knees and standing up into water fall forward bend. Folding from your hips, allow the head to hang as you surrender the neck. You may bend your knees to ensure the back is relaxed. Feel all four corners of the feet in the earth, especially into the front balls of the feet next to the big toe. Do not lean into the heels too much. Relax in this position as you continue a smooth rhythm of a flowing breathes.

17. Crescent Moon Pose – from Waterfall Forward Bend Pose. (Repeat of # 15) Repeat the Crescent Moon Pose now on the other side. Bend your knees and move the right leg back behind you. Place your right knee in the ground as pictured above. Move your left leg in front of you with bent knee. Left foot should be easily resting fully in the ground flat on the sole. The heel of the left foot is under the right knee on the floor. You are in a lunge position. Inhale while moving the torso upward to the sky and stretching the spine. Open the chest and heart center as you

reach your arms behind you, each inhale reaching your heart up and each exhale releasing deeper into your bend. Enjoy how you feel as you continue your ujayii breathing in this expansive pose. Reach the heart towards the moon. Complete three sets of breathes or more.

18. Cat Pose (Repeat of #6) – repeat the Cat Pose, now from the Crescent Moon. Move your torso forward onto your hands and knees and arch your back upward toward the sun. As you exhale, press your belly up into your spine.

19. Camel Pose – from Cat Pose, use the abdominals and lift torso up to kneeling position. Bend elbows and bring hands into lower back with palms facing in. Elbows bent. You can remain here if you like in a back bend with elbows moving gently behind you toward each other. Inhale the spine upward, exhale the head back if it is comfortable for neck. Open the heart center upward. Gently press your hips forward. To go deeper into this back bend, straighten the arms behind you and reach and clasp heels of

feet. You can choose to keep your feet flat or for easier reach fold your toes inward. Breathe in and out as many breaths as you like opening the heart center deeply.

20. Open Heart Seal Pose – from Camel pose, inhale head upward to stretch the spine again. Now fold forward from the hips sitting onto your feet. The feet should be flat. Gently relax your forehead onto the floor or onto a folded towel or Yoga block just make sure you relax your head, neck and shoulders. Rest your arms and hands on the ground by your sides. Slowly bring your hands together into your lower back and inter lace your fingers together. Your palms are facing each other as you begin to lift your arms up off of your back either keeping your elbows bent or straightening them as you like. Breathe big into your chest keeping head and neck relaxed. Allow the hips and legs and feet to melt into the ground as you exhale and repeat three sets of breaths.

21. Fish Pose – moving out of the Open Heart Seal Pose, release the arms into the floor beside your hips. Slowly sit up onto

your feet with your buttocks. Use your abdominals and arms to lower yourself onto your back. Bring your arms and shoulder blades toward each other under your back while lifting the whole back off the floor. Keep your buttocks and legs on the ground. Use your arms and bend your elbows to assist you. Now, allow your head to move backward as the top of your head reaches for the ground as you slide your torso further back lengthening your spine and arms. The crown of the head will rest gently on the ground or a towel or blanket. The crown is the top of the head, not the back of head. Inhale chest and heart center up toward the sky, as you exhale pressing out stale air out from your lungs while you power out through your abdominals and pelvic and base of the spine muscles assisting you in releasing the air in order to create space to drink in the new clean air to the lungs. Create the "haaahh" sound each time you exhale. Bring more new air in with each inhale through the nose. Continue to open your heart center more and then some more allowing the heart to soften and become light. Complete three sets of breaths or more.

22. Supine Spinal Twist – release slowly out of Fish pose and rest comfortably onto your back, lightly tucking the chin forward toward the chest. Relax the head into the floor. Bring your knees into your chest for a deep back stretch. Follow by crossing your left leg over your right thigh. Open the arms away from each other and out to the sides and move your knees slowly to the right side. Now, rest feet and knees on the floor and allow them to melt into the ground. Take a slow, deep breathe in. Then release your breath as you close your eyes and feel the movement of air flowing through your body. Feel your body release into this twist. Look toward your left arm the best you can gently stretching your neck. Take as many breaths as needed. When you have gotten what you need from this side, engage the core center to begin moving back into a neutral spine and move into the other side. Continue your conscious breathing, feeling the ebb and flow of your breath moving in your body assisting you and releasing deeper

into you asana. Relax your neck and head. Here, take another slow, deep breath for however long you desire.

23. Corpse, or Relaxation Pose – use the strength of your core center to move slowly out of the Spinal Twist Pose. Now is the time—ONLY AFTER YOU HAVE A TEACHER—to put on your oxygen headset for final pose and meditation. Relax onto your back. Take a big, deep wonderful breath in and a slow, long beautiful exhale with a "haaahh" sound to release any toxins and tension from the body, mind and spirit. Gently tuck the chin in toward the chest then release. Move the shoulders softly down toward the hands. Slide the hips down toward the feet. Close the eyes, let go of your head, neck and shoulders. Relax your arms, back and hips. Feel your right leg being massaged by the earth, and now your left leg too. Allow your feet and hands to spread open and then relax them. Your breath now is resting along with your body. Truly let go and surrender here and now.

Congratulations!

You have taken your first journey into Oxygen Yoga. Rest here as you reap the benefits and allow yourself to receive whatever your being needs at this moment in time.

Remember that an Oxygen Yoga teacher is required to help you get true benefit and results from your efforts. **AND, NEVER USE OXYGEN WITHOUT A TRAINED PROFESSIONAL GUIDING YOU EVERY TIME YOU PRACTICE THE POSES** OR UNTIL YOU BECOME PROFICENT. You must know how to use the oxygen safely.

Use the *Oxygen Yoga Pure & Simple textbook* to study the poses via the photographs in full color and to find your teacher. Practice these poses at least three times a week for eight weeks per cycle to gain best results. During your practice learn to consciously open your heart to unconditional love and peace of the universe. The ideal time to meditate is shortly after a set of poses has been practiced. This is the time when the mind and body are most relaxed and prepared to focus. You can also meditate without practicing the asana at any time you choose. We do recommend that you meditate every day for about twenty minutes at any time that is convenient for you. There are actual meditations in the textbook that have proven to be helpful.

We want to hear from you. Please visit www.oxygenyogabook.com for more information. E-mail your comments or opinions to oxygenyoga@gmail.com

CHAPTER 7

THE PROMISE OF A BODY FULL OF OXYGEN

From the time we were that marvelous infant, that child we can all still feel and sometimes re-connect with, lying there in the cradle, taking in the awe-inspiring input from our environment, our minds have constantly formed their connection with the universe—on the one hand gulping data, and on the other learning to put it into action.

As we did then, we still interpret the environment around us in our own unique ways. We are creating the world now, just as we were then—and, we continue with this masterful pursuit as we mature and even as we pass on into the next realm. From the octogenarian's point of view, the visual impact of the world around them is still a miracle of sensory input as it was when the mature person was a child.

* * *OGA NOTE * * *

With the extremely obnoxious stressors that surround us, that we endure endlessly, there is no simple fix like fight or flight. It is good when necessary. If we are pumped up, and there is no need to fight or flight, then our bodies are pooling this energy, so we need another outlet. If we really don't have to run or fight, our physical body doesn't get to react—society does not even allow it. We hold in penned up energy that is ready to explode. Our conscious mind and physical self is overridden with this flood of adrenaline rushing through us, but we simply have to endure the stressors. This enormous physical tension causes us to react internally, producing today's diseases.

This bind of the modern person can be very well soothed with Oxygen Yoga. As we feel into our bodies, get stretched out, enhance self awareness, we can learn to relax out of any annoyance and let it slide right off.

Looking out on the miracle of being, centenarians do not immediately notice the aging of the body they are in—the outward environment feels completely fresh and new in its reality. Since the very roots of today's understanding: philosophers, savants, metaphysicians, great thinkers have shared points of convergence in relationship to the understanding of how we work with information.

The child in the cradle gathers, processes, assigns level of importance, of usability and produces a masterpiece of an image for use in the moment, storage, and retrieval. This entire process is entirely entwined with all of the energies commingling throughout the universe. Our ocular, nasal, hearing, the skin itself, all of the fantastic sensing devices work with minute data and assemble them into entire structures, panoramas, the sweep and majesty of the heavens. We sense our interconnectedness with the largest spectrum.

And to add to the miracle, we can pull little bits and pieces of vast images out, view them like a photo album or even relive them in slow motion. Then, as casually as if we were brushing our teeth, we tuck this intricate data away for later retrieval. Our minds are amazingly agile, dazzling in their speed and accuracy, unfathomable in their complexity, unbelievably trustworthy, and arranged in a fabulous weave of magical quality. They mix with our immediate environment and extend on, out into the heavens in a multiplexing event that is beyond belief. That is basically how it works until stress, in any form, comes into play.

Today, in our toxin-laced, accelerated culture various forces like mental tension from a harsh, crammed environment join with others, like carbon monoxide and airborne particulates. These ramparts of stress effect our minds severely. Our wonderful systems are endowed with numerous tools for working with this toxic buffet. Our minds and bodies are truly religious in nature—that is, they operate from the sense of devotion related to any truly religious act. They work beautifully in a vast continuum of change. One of the great blessings of the universe is the fabulous gift of our minds. The great challenge is to drop all the discursive thinking jammed into us through the years, so we can learn how to use it to its fullest. We are born relating to the world with our full, instinctive knowledge, but as we grow and absorb the sordid, defective thinking so often promoted in our everyday environment many of us lose our freshness.

Oxygen Yoga has been developed to regain that vitality in our lives. We need to relax into meditation, into the mantra of oxygen-plentiful breathing, and be re-merged with the fine tuning of the brain's unlimited abilities. The mind is the center of the entire being as it encompasses one's intellect, imagination, creativity, thoughts and feelings. Therefore, paying close attention to and caring for it are crucial in maintaining a state of overall well being, mentally as well as emotionally and physically.

THE UNFOLDING OF THE OGA PATH

- You, the new practitioner read this handbook for the basics.
- You see that corporate pollution has robbed you of your birthright to O_2.
- The new practitioner works with the poses that are in the textbook in large full color.
- The novitiate is deeply intrigued by the promise of O_2 moving in through her lungs and out through the blood stream to every nook and cranny of her body which is oxygen starved.
- The novitiate takes the primal step and engages a teacher
- The amazing 20% mix of O_2 is experienced with an "Ah Ha! This is it. Something I have known but never felt."

- The novitiate begins working regularly with the teacher and feels a profound chain of new understanding throughout life.

The experience of witnessing the unfolding of our minds is limitless. The limitations are those that we place on our own selves learned from defective fear-based teaching in our youths—most times we are not even aware that we are actually not living to our full potential. We all have our own unique, special interpretation of the world we live in and the ability to express ourselves in a myriad of wonderful ways.

Each strand and fiber of the great universal whole has a special purpose on this earth. The brain is known as the direct communicator, the integration facilitator for the body as a whole. It communicates freely with every organ and body part. When one engages fully in Oxygen Yoga postures and Oxygen Meditation, the past, present and future can converge, melding as the experience of timelessness, of the ego disappearing into the here and now, the totality of the never ending moment. There is a particular climactic period during Oxygen Meditation when aging can actually stop. With the training, the brain increases its ability to communicate with body parts right down to the cellular level—and then on down to the molecular level where communication changes take place and slow the pace of aging momentarily. During this moment of the cessation of aging that one encounters during the meditative state, one can discover Self, the Universe and one's own, unique Purpose and Position in relationship to all else. This discovery promotes peace within the individual by removing those same undesirable forces, which promote early aging. The goal is for the practitioner to learn to flow through life in a more joyful and content existence. This occurs naturally and the individual learns their true value by connecting to the unconditional love of the Creator of their own being and of all things. It is stated in Psalm 46:10: Be still, and know that I am God.

* * * OGA NOTE * * *

What Is Oxygen Meditation and What Are the Benefits?

Oxygen Meditation is a form for attainment of deep mind opening through concentration on a fixed object, the oxygen molecule. It is a connection to the universe. During the process, the individual can see themselves as an integral part of the entire universe. Each

strand and fiber of the great universal whole has a special purpose on this earth.

Since thoughts have a direct impact on physical and emotional feelings, it stands to reason that practicing meditation is essential for a positive and substantial life. There are different levels of meditation and the goal in Oxygen Meditation is to allow oneself to meld with our natural, universal state of deep peace.

The brain is known as the direct communicator, the integration facilitator for the body as a whole. It communicates freely with every organ and body part. When one engages fully in Yoga postures before Oxygen Meditation, the past, present and future can converge, melting as the experience of timelessness, of the ego disappearing into the here and now, the totality of the never ending moment.

While connected with Unconditional Love and becoming aware of the universal embrace, one can enjoy a sense of complete security and the illumination of all the fine qualities of the connected self. As we unite with our higher self, our spirit, we enjoy a delicious reprieve from the ongoing banter of ego's struggle to maintain our outward personality—what is often referred to as the self. This is not the true self. The experience of the quietness of Unconditional Love is our actual self. It is soft and flowing. The false self is ego's striving to maintain stasis, the need for which arises from fear.

In an amazingly prompt series of awakenings, the magnificent intake of a proper balance of oxygen will instigate your feeling more in touch with yourself and your purpose on this earth. As you get to know your true self, your inner self in a deeper way, you will become aware of your purpose. You will become aware of the pre-programmed wiring of instinct and your protective and survival mechanisms. This is not social conditioning—you weren't taught these native understandings, you were born with them. It has all been pre-coded for you. These abilities and more are truly innate, like birds flying south.

As the negative thoughts and the inhibitions that keep you from your authentic self float out of your being, you can lighten up, and relax into the genuine, more peaceful person that is actually you. The struggle of life will soon lessen and peace and joy will overcome you. Think oxygen! Letting the mind go and explore such vibrant and free thoughts, can help to clear it of any stress and worries that everyday life may bring upon you. The mind will feel refreshed and rejuvenated. This journey into Oxygen Meditation can help invoke a light hearted feeling at any time simply by thinking back to the general lightness of being experienced during each session of your practice. When the mind feels relaxed and clear, the body too, will feel rejuvenated. Thus, reiterating the idea that the well-being of the mind has a direct effect on the well-being of the entire body. We have the ability to do this by strengthening the mind through meditation and practicing changing our thoughts.

CHAPTER 8

TODAY IS SPA DAY

Human beings are without choice—the intake of a healthy, clean and reliable source of oxygen must be there throughout our lives. Not only is oxygen an absolute necessity for keeping us alive; it is one of the most vital elements for health and beauty: and, it is an absolute joy to feel it work with one's being.

* * * OGA NOTE * * *

Since disease-causing bacteria and viruses are nearly all anaerobic, meaning that they cannot survive in an oxygenated environment, a medium rich in O_2 can promote a vital sense of well-being and the

mending of our damaged bodies. These attributes that the use of oxygen brings make it a much sought-after tool for use in spas and beauty facilities.

It is so powerful and diverse in the healing and restoration of healthy skin that it has become common-place in spa regimens, and very highly touted in home facial products as well. Oxygen facials, for example, infuse the skin with the wonderful molecules, bringing its benefits right to the skin cells. Over and over again, it is used with the beautifying and preservation of the epidermis, even combined into treatments like micro-derm abrasion, but the magic is that it is not like some corporate-sales hype, some silly vanity—no, the body understands the deep connection with our primal, universal being as we relax into Oxygen Yoga.

The need for the support of O_2 is super important in this day and age. Global warming; the lack of shielding for UV rays in our atmosphere; and the toxic cocktail that our ambient air has turned into from automobiles and industry: all combined with urban stress and an accelerated culture, contribute without leniency to horrid wear and tear on our bodies.

The symptoms compound daily: dry, irritated skin; billions of people with epidermal tissue that has been grossly damaged by the sun; waves of skin problems such as acne, clogged pores and cancers. All of the complaints are well suited for the O2 treatments.

And the ghastly pounding of our spirits from the grasping mentality inculcated into us by corporate marketing—melting into Oxygen Yoga stills the spirit quickly because it is so grounding. New and amazing pathways to renovation and rejuvenation of the skin, of all the body, and the promotion of robust potency and vigor with it open continuously. Simply breathing oxygen into the lungs can improve health and relieve pain—both spiritual and physical. Doing Oxygen Yoga we breathe deeply and oxygen is restored to the body tissues faster. If we have a real supply of O_2, rather than the filthy air in our cities, our bodies can really be supplied well. The vigorous intake of a healthy mix is the obvious reason that Oxygen Yoga can do so much for the practitioner.

THE WONDER OF OXYGEN – OUR BODIES REQUIRE IT FOR SO MANY TASKS

- Respiration
- Healing of wounds
- Detoxification of our bodies
- Reduction of inflammation
- Strengthening of the skin's elasticity
- Collagen
- Providing a healthy antibacterial environment for cells

Wondrous little joys like touching up the fine lines can produce that fresh, youthful appearance to the neck and face. The healthy look for which so many very-old Yogins and Yoginis in clean-air locations are so well known begin to make themselves available.

These small treasures can be a fabulous addition to one's life: Treating the epidermis when toxicity effects it at an early age, working with the body in clearing up pore infections like pimples, helping cure the damages from our depleted Ozone layer. As the novitiate surrounds herself with the wonders of O_2, she will discover the surprising amount of attention that our oxygen supply is getting now with all the new interest in environmental issues.

For example, the reader will discover that oxygen can be delivered to their door. Massage therapists have been known to make a visit to the home with their portable units to do massage. It is stored in tanks of varying sizes, from just a fraction of a liter to several liters. The smaller units are portable, and can be administered as inhaled oxygen, oxygen mist, or even as facial treatments like the Oxygen Spa Facial System. Oxygen for beauty and anti-aging benefits is extremely popular because of its proven effectiveness. One of the more common ways to deliver oxygen for anti-aging benefits is directly to the skin in the form of an oxygenated cream or through Oxygen Therapy in which oxygen is infused into the skin. Oxygen facials enhance the skin's firmness and youthfulness and oxygenate the skin at a cellular level for an Oxygen Facelift. The great power of this treatment is that a lack of oxygen causes the skin to age prematurely and supplying oxygen to the skin can restore the wonderful, original texture of one's epidermis.

* * * OGA NOTE * * *

The need for the support of O_2 is super important in this day and age. Global warming; the lack of shielding for UV rays

in our atmosphere; and the toxic cocktail
that our ambient air has turned into from
automobiles and industry: all combined
with urban stress and an Accelerated culture,
contribute without leniency to horrid wear
and tear on our bodies.

The symptoms compound daily: dry, irritated
skin; billions of people with epidermal
tissue that has been grossly damaged by the
sun; waves of skin problems such as acne or
clogged pores. All of the complaints are well
suited for the O_2 treatments. And the horrid
pounding of our spirits from the grasping
mentality inculcated into us by corporate
marketing—melting into Oxygen Yoga stills
the spirit quickly because it is so grounding.

Package, contain liquid oxygen in order
to treat the skin as it is being cleaned and
moisturized. These products can really work
with the aging process, remove particulates
from the ambient air, scrub up, hydrate, and
rebalance all in one process. One of our favorite
product lines is the Oxygenated Ajna cleaners
and creams with nutrients by Bella Lumen
Labs. These products are phenomenal. They all
enhance the Oxygen Yoga practitioner's sense
of well being, and with the grounding of the

meditation bring forth a rebirth in contact with our sacred centers. The amazing gas can also be infused into water through an oxygenator, and the individual receiving treatment can soak in the infused water.

One of the more effective ways to deliver oxygen is via a hyperbaric oxygen chamber, a device that surrounds the body creating pressurized oxygen that forces the healing gas into the tissues. Hyperbaric chambers are used in hospitals as well as spas for miraculous, uplifting treatments like wound and burn healing, skin graft healing, and rejuvenation therapies. Hyperbaric applications use the monoplace and multiplace units. The mono equipment is easier on the pocket book and more compact. The mono equipment also requires less training.

Multiplace chambers can be very impacting, but a trained specialist is required to administer the treatment. Inaccurate treatment of gas pressure is a strict taboo. New equipment comes to the market each day as we continue to unravel the vast importance of O_2 for all living creatures. Ozonators charge spa water and fight organisms rather than using chemicals. Machines such as the oxygen delivery systems provide safe, effective and non-invasive delivery of oxygen to the skin.

There is a reason and exactness for everything on this earth and in the universe. Everything has been created and did not just happen; genes have been precisely programmed in certain ways that we don't always understand. The "origins of life" is a vast subject, which no one yet has been able to scientifically prove. It is mysterious. During your meditation, think about the vastness of the universe and our purpose here on earth. It will make all of us better, kinder and more caring people who are in tune with our surroundings. As the scriptures have it, love other as you love yourself. Love your environment that you have been so carefully placed in. Open your mind to all that surrounds and you will find the answers to your questions. This powerful, holistic application of Oga will send the Practioner home feeling better, looking younger, and enjoying better health. All of those mechanics are important. They bring one into the moment, into a true enjoyment of our lives. And, they can readily cause us to meld with the calm dignity of our path, our natural Spiritual Way.

RAISING WIND HORSE

Taking the reins of Wind Horse is a Tibetan expression for raising our energy to its zenith. Just like Oxygen Yoga, we use the breath, to raise wind horse. We empty the mind and become totally at one with the moment. We forget about goals and ambitions. We forget about Enlightenment. We chuck Spiritual Paths and The Way right out the window and lose our ego within whatever we are doing. We become the eternal, never ending moment and at long last know exactly who we are.

If you have skipped from the front of the Handbook and want to join us for the new, 21st Century fast-tracking to enlightenment, follow your intuition, get on line at <u>www.</u>

<u>oxygenyogabook.com</u>. You will need a copy of *Oxygen Yoga Pure & Simple textbook* and to begin taking all the courses and using the tapes. You will quickly find your mind melting away, the oxygen flooding your lungs, the Yoga wrapping you up in a blanket of calm that you have never experienced. As you read *Oxygen Yoga Pure & Simple*, textbook you will meld with the photos and open to the amazing new world of 21st Century Paths to brilliant and very rapid Enlightened Mind.

Oxygen Yoga is also referred to as OGA (o-ga), a brief snappy term for people on the move who are quickly making it one of the most sought after classes in the entire 21st Century to take. It is about exercising in the cleanest air possible and to give your body the full advantage of the movements. Dirt, dust, germs, smog and allergens are all things we want to avoid. Bringing clean fresh oxygen to the brain helps improve clarity. You will notice the difference the moment you start.

After reading the Handbook, you will move right into the Textbook. Order *Oxygen Yoga Pure & Simple* quickly on the net at www. oxygenyogabook.com, and check the resource page in the back of the book. You will be wise to start classes as soon as you receive the book. Classes for beginners and certification classes for instructors can also be found in the back of the book.

Using the oxygen that is missing in your life as you relax into the grounded movements of Oxygen Yoga automatically begins to open the mind. "Oga," as described in this Handbook and elucidated further in the textbook—*Oxygen Yoga Pure & Simple*—will prove to be a wonderful way to open your entire being further and further. As you open, you will notice a marked new sense of relaxation. In the textbook you will find some meditations to practice to begin your deep meditations and your journey to calm centered self.

If you have already studied Yoga, you will appreciate that this practice is an effective addition to your current practice. The body craves oxygen, and once it feels a proper balance you will be pleasantly surprised. As you begin to take the courses you will use *Oxygen Yoga Pure & Simple* as your guide. That is why it should be ordered right away—once your heart, your soul, your lungs, and your starving mind feel the input of oxygen, you will not want to delay your experience.

Another reason for ordering *Oxygen Yoga Pure & Simple* immediately is that you will find your certified instructor in the information section at the back of the volume. You will require the hands-on guidance of a certified instructor. Many people enjoy the use of oxygen to clear their minds, but it is essential that you remember that you are seriously altering the body's supply of the substance that is most vital for its well being. Never undertake such critical acts in a cavalier manner.

This handbook will engage your interest and point you in the right direction. As your interest grows you will see how important it is to be careful with your methods of oxygen intake. You will need your instructor, your classes and *Oxygen Yoga Pure & Simple* ASAP. Please be certain to take the time to learn how to use equipment before purchasing it. Keep in mind at all times that, although it can be an extremely enjoyable situation to feel your bloodstream bathed in oxygen, a part of your supply is not coming from the air around you. Anything stored under pressure in a tank must be handled with care and with the advice of experts, so start with the information in the back of *Oxygen Yoga Pure & Simple textbook* and open the doors to a brand new life. The textbook is available worldwide.

If you are considering taking the instructor course, you should already be a yoga instructor, or at least, a certified trainer. As we have explained, the textbook and study guide—which is necessary for the class—is available on line and in bookstores. For all of you who decide to become certified in

Oga, remember that to avoid delay, you need to buy the books before arriving at the class.

This Handbook gives that always handy overview, a basic introduction and understanding of Oga. Then, the textbook takes you into the work much more deeply. It provides fabulous, inspirational illustrations and photography. Not only are the graphics an aid to learning; they provide a never ending inspirational boost similar to that of a breath of fresh, well oxygenated air.

The full color Oxygen Yoga textbook has been chosen with care for the spiritual enlivening we receive from color. It contains many enlarged illustrations, which enhance learning the poses and using your oxygen tools correctly. *Oxygen Yoga Pure & Simple* will springboard you on from this Handbook, helping you move quickly, coaching you on, into the correct mindset for using Oxygen equipment.

The equipment is only for individuals who are already certified and people enrolled in an approved class. To find out if an instructor is certified in your area, check in the book or contact www.oxygenyogabook.com. Always beware of untrained and authorized people teaching classes. It is always best to check with us, the originators of "Oxygen Yoga" before engaging in the classes to avoid any danger.

Doing "Oga" is an art form and requires special ability in developing breathing skills, movements and meditations. All instructors must have exacting training for teaching students how to safely maximize their experience. It is also important to come to the realization that not every person is receptive to this type of training.

For instance, a person who has been practicing a particular form of yoga for many years may not be as receptive as a new generation of "Oga's." Sometimes a person can get stuck in habit and develop the perception that there is only one way to perform yoga. If you are an instructor who can easily adapt to changes in your present understanding of yoga, you will readily see that oxygen is a marvelous enhancement to an ancient tradition and immediately become a candidate for this program.

As with all things in the world, we are growing and changing all the time. Nothing ever stands still unless we learn to and wake up and step outside the stress of time and open up the here and now. Be still in the moment. We learn more and more as specialists and all sorts of professionals realize the great potential of enjoying a healthy life style.

If you are a Chiropractor, you may want to consider Oga for helping to align the spine and improve posture. Oga is a great way to help people breath properly and stand up straight. It causes people to get involved in their own health. It is also great for senior citizens with other problems. It is an easy way for them to exercise with out feeling fatigued. Most Chiropractors enjoy holding the classes because it brings people together and increases business.

Esthicians can implement the "Oga" into their facial programs. Simply allow the person to wear the headset and rotate their limbs to help the person fully relax. Esthicians have done mediations with the client to get them to loosen up, to help bring circulation back into the face, while providing the much needed oxygen to the skin. In the future it will be a must have for all day spas.

Massage therapists can take the equipment with them to provide oxygen meditation while massaging their client and helping them get centered. It is a wonderful way to help them relax.

Doctor's offices can supply oxygen to the patients while they are in the waiting room to help them relax and not mind the waiting time. They will endure the will go through the wait with enjoyment and be tickled to return for more.

Gyms and other training facilities cannot afford to be without this program and equipment. You will need to send someone to get certified. It is not just enough to learn about oxygen, but to understand the entire Oga philosophy. It is about bringing people along mentally, giving them the base from which they can enjoy the full effects of exercise and really get strong and want to return without urging because Oga makes life easier—they can feel it. This is the future; it's time to get ready for it by enrolling in one of our week-end get-a-ways.

It only takes one week-end to get the basic certification and begin your Oga practice. It will be a lovely and beneficial experience, and be prepared to get in touch with the universe and yourself. Hope to see you there. The certification classes are held across the country.

Destin and Panama City Beach are choice locations because of the pristine and protected white beaches. Purity at its utmost! Even if you are not able to take the classes or week-end retreats consider exploring this particular area in the Gulf of Mexico. And please, watch out for our next book, coming soon.

This is a call to the reader to join us all in the new wave, the avant-garde of environmental, spiritual, physical presence and understanding that is sweeping the planet

So you can now pick up this handbook and as soon as you realize what a profoundly important document you have stumbled across, you will want to order your own copy of, The *Oxygen Yoga Pure & Simple,* textbook and find the nearest workshops. Stop living in your mind and feel the depth of this unforgettable work, this most amazing of experiences and bring your entire being back to life by nurturing your body with it's most primordial, most basic and most required substance—fresh, clean oxygen.

This avant-garde, this new wave of moving directly into the Enlightened Mind is full of the most noble twists of fate and the convergence of the greatest of all our amazing history of teachers: Jesus, Buddha, Gandhi, Dali Lama, Baha'u'llah, and others, practicing non-violent work. Peace is the only answer for the success of the human population; otherwise we will make ourselves extinct. That is our only choice. Chaos is what we have in many cities today and is the beginning of the end of our world as we know it unless we find a way to stop it. It is so important to be aware and pay attention to what is happening to us and our planet. How far will it all go? Where are our limits as human beings? Peace is also another word for love and hate is another word for fear.

The myriad teachings have opened up from the East for re-birth and re-invigoration in the

West; massive opening of the ancient knowledge of attending to the temple of our bodies.

This spiritual path is one of great power and this fantastic new wave does not swerve away from the old verities. If one takes a look at a magazine like *What is Enlightenment*, it is absolutely powerful to see that such a profound question is being discussed in the open, no-holds-barred, precisely, clearly and right up front for us one and all.

Oxygen Yoga is one of the key components of the 21st Century path to understanding. As you read *Oxygen Yoga Pure & Simple*, you will feel compelled to stop missing out on life and to join the flow. It's time to move on, to get absorbed in the book and get hooked on oxygen & Yoga both. This miracle is our step forward, our sacred offering to our readers, a Path toward taking the reins away from television, pills, junk food, speed and aggression. It provides a method for slowing down, zeroing in on ourselves, practicing actual full breathing and stepping through the portal of renewed energy, back into a vital life.

"A heart at peace gives life to the body"

Proverbs 14:30

ABOUT THE AUTHORS

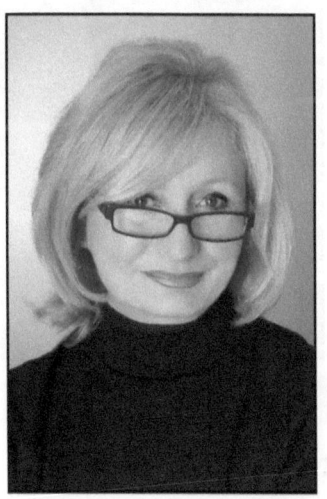

Barbara has a graduate degree as a chemist. She believes that the world was designed by an intelligent creator and that we are all products the grand design. She is a proponent of world peace and education. As a humanitarian, she is currently writing on human cruelty and hatred with the hopes of presenting a better understanding and promoting peace. As a writer she has appeared on television, radio and has made public appearances for the platforms described. As a scientist she is involved in the study of aging, health and beauty industries.

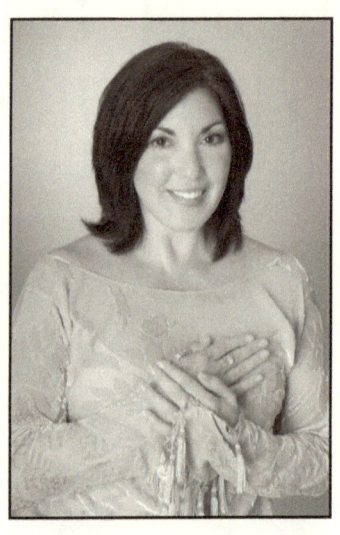

Lisa, a certified Yoga teacher, has been actively pursuing "The Philosophy of Life" and mental peace within the universe. She has incorporated this quest for knowledge and her passion for health and wellness by teaching individuals and groups at various high profile locations thought out New York and Connecticut. Her interest in imagery and hypnosis, ayurvedic therapy, flower essences, aroma therapy, physiology and anatomy has led her to various forms of yoga, culminating in her own version of relaxation techniques, which maximize the yoga experience with Oxygen Yoga. She is currently researching and experimenting with the mind-body connection and the innovative use of color in conjunction with various forms of exercise for mental optimization, ultimate vitality and longevity.

www.ingramcontent.com/pod-product-compliance
Lightning Source LLC
Chambersburg PA
CBHW020254290526
45784CB00003B/1244
9781438912769